# Intermittent Fasting

## *The Essential Beginners Guide for Women for Weight Loss*

**LELA GIBSON**

# CONTENTS

# Introduction

I want to thank you and congratulate you for buying the book, *"Intermittent Fasting: the Essential Beginners Guide for Women for Weight Loss"*.

This book has lots of actionable information on how, as a woman, you can unleash the full power of intermittent fasting for weight loss.

Struggling to lose weight, and repeatedly failing at it, has to be one of the most soul-crushing things any of us could ever experience especially so for women. This is especially so for women since the general perception of an ideal body that defines beauty, health and happiness of a woman revolves around her body shape that is heavily impacted by weight.

Body fat gets packed in different places for both sexes; a man will rarely ever have to struggle with stubborn fat in the upper arms, for instance, while a woman who gains a few pounds will certainly face the prospect of burning upper arm fat that just refuses to go. While men do gain fat in the 'love handles' area, their case is rarely as bad as that of women.

Out there, in the vast universe that is the internet, are countless diets and workout programs targeting belly fat, which is the cause of worry for most men. Comparably, very few programs target the body fat woes of women. Most men can fight body fat using a combination of diet and building lean muscle. Unfortunately, it is harder for women given that muscle gain, lean or not, is not an attractive option for most.

In relation to shedding body fat, intermittent fasting (also known as IF) is revolutionary. Think about it; what other method promises you to lose weight without a list of 'eat this not that' and some other set of impossible to follow rules? IF prides in one major thing - allowing its adopter, more so women, to drop stubborn body fat without the usual rigor that comes with 'special diets'. It also impacts on beauty and wholeness of any human in a major way.

This book will walk you through how, as a woman, you can adopt intermittent fasting to torch fat deposited at various points of the body without gaining any lean muscles.

Thanks again for buying this book. I hope you enjoy it!

Before we get to a point of discussing how to follow intermittent fasting as a woman to attain maximum weight loss, let's start by building a strong understanding of the concept of intermittent fasting.

# Intermittent Fasting: A Comprehensive Understanding

A resounding question that might be ringing in your mind right now is - what in the world is intermittent fasting? Let me answer that:

**What is it?**

In its simplest terms, intermittent fasting is deciding that you will skip some (specific) meals. In simple terms, when following intermittent fasting, you fast and follow the fast by eating on purpose. Well, you don't stay away from food altogether, as is the case with starvation, before going back to your normal eating habits. Rather, you target specific 'windows' during your days to eat after holding your fast.

By fasting and then following it with feasting on purpose, fasting intermittently means you eat your calories during a special window or windows in your day, and make the choice not to eat during the rest of the day.

To put it in simpler terms, it entails fasting during a specific interval 'time block' then feasting in the next interval. A classic example of this type of fasting interval is; fasting for 24 hours then resuming normal eating for the next 24 hours. You go on like this, 24 hours intervals, until the desired results – weight loss, low food craving - are realized. Another classic one is breakfast to breakfast fasting, then breakfast to breakfast feasting and doing it for as long as possible or necessary. That means; on day 1, you skip any eating between the time you wake up in the morning and supper but take supper. On day 2, resume normal eating and repeat the cycle (repeat fasting) on day 3, followed by fasting on day 4.

## What Is the Point Of All This?

This works on several fronts. By shutting yourself from food most of the day, which is what intermittent fasting will call for, you limit the amount of calories you consume. A lower intake of calories means there is less for the body to turn into body fat (the body converts excess calories to fats).

Let me explain that in detail:

When you eat food (especially the carb rich diet that's recommended by USDA i.e. the typical American diet), it is broken down into different components depending on the macronutrients you've eaten. Fats are converted into fatty acids, proteins are converted into amino acids and carbohydrates are converted into glucose. All these are absorbed into the bloodstream for transportation to different parts of the body. When they get into the bloodstream, the body is triggered to secrete insulin a hormone produced by the pancreas. The role of insulin in this case is to sort of open up the cells so that they can take up various macronutrients for energy. It does this by increasing the cells' affinity to micronutrients. Glucose, which tends to be high in the typical American diet has the highest effect on the amount of insulin secreted. Typically, the higher the blood glucose levels, the higher the amount of insulin produced.

You are in the fed state from the moment you start eating to the time the body to the time the body uses up all the food you've taken. This can take anywhere between 10-12 hours. The fed state is however categorized into two; the fed state i.e. which starts from the moment you start eating and lasts for about 3-5 hours from the last meal and the post absorption state, a state where the body is actively using up the nutrients you have taken and lasts for about 10-12 hours from the last meal. During the fed state, insulin levels are high because of elevated levels of blood sugar. Keep in mind that insulin is secreted in response to rising blood glucose levels and decreases as blood glucose levels reduce. As I already stated, insulin does the job of aiding blood glucose into the cells. Its job essentially is to trigger the cells to 'open up' so that they can absorb glucose; insulin acts like a key to the cells to let blood glucose into the cells. This essentially means that if there is any excess blood glucose, insulin will still trigger the cells to absorb the glucose.

If there is any excess, the body (the liver) starts by converting it to glycogen, which is then stored in the liver and muscle cells. Glycogen stores are however limited so the body has to find a place to store the excess. Fats are the other method through which the body stores excess glucose. Essentially, the glucose is converted into fatty acids and glycerol, which are then stored in different fat stores around the body e.g. under the skin and around various internal organs. The whole process takes place within 10-12 hours so once the hours lapse, the body will essentially have used up all the glucose from the bloodstream.

This is when it gets into the fasted state, a state where the body has no incoming dietary nutrients that it can use for energy. When that happens, it starts mobilizing its stored energy as it awaits any new dietary nutrients. It starts by secreting glucagon from the pancreas to help convert glycogen into glucose, which is then used just like dietary glucose. However, it doesn't metabolize all the glycogen before moving on to fats; it still needs some glucose to fuel critical cell activities that run on glucose only. As such, when you get into the fasted state, you slowly start burning stored fats to meet your body's energy demands. This is what results to weight loss.

This means that if you want to derive benefits from intermittent fasting, you ought to fast for long enough to get your body into the fasted state, as this will push the body to seek alternative sources of energy e.g. burning stored fat.

As you continue with intermittent fasting, your body gets to a point where it is adapted to using smaller amounts of food (unless you go all out during the feasting window, you are unlikely to consume the same amount of food that you have been eating. This essentially pushes your body to be more efficient in utilizing various nutrients and helps you to have an easy time in switching to healthy food. This can in turn enable you to derive the benefits of healthy eating.

So what's the best way to fast intermittently? Here are ideas:

**Eat at specific times:** For instance, you can skip breakfast and schedule your meals in a way that allows you to eat from noon to 8 PM. Such an 8-hour window will see you skip breakfast altogether to maintain it. If taking a full 24-hour break is difficult, skip 2 meals on some days. If handling a specific eating window is a bit difficult and your only option is to follow the regular eating schedule that sees you finish dinner at 8 PM, you can stay away from eating again on some days until 8 PM the next day.

We will discuss more of how to fast intermittently in a later chapter.

**Note:** The body tends to react to energy consumption (eating food) with the production of insulin. Essentially, the more your body is sensitive to insulin, the more likely it is that it will use what food you consume efficiently. This will help you lose weight. Along with this, your body will be most sensitive to insulin immediately following a fasting period. Your glycogen levels will greatly reduce during your fasting period, and will deplete to an even further degree when exercising, which spikes up your insulin sensitivity.

By focusing on specific feeding windows, and getting your body used to them, your body will adapt itself so that it 'expects' a feeding during these windows; this will optimize the process of burning up food to form energy.

The same will go for exercising in a fasted state. If you choose to go in this direction (and you really should, if you are really keen on losing body fat), without a readily available glucose or glycogen supply to burn, as it has been depleted over the duration of your fast without replenishment, your body has no choice but to adapt. It has to pull from the one energy source available, which is the fat stored in your cells.

What we've learnt so far is an overall understanding of intermittent fasting, which applies to both men and women.

# Intermittent Fasting For Women: What You Need To Know

The question you might have is; so how exactly can you follow intermittent fasting as a woman? Well, compared to men, women experience intermittent fasting quite differently. It is, a lot of the time, trickier for a woman to get results. The weight and psychological benefits are still possible but as a woman, you may have to approach the process differently.

From the previous paragraph, it is clear why you may have to approach the process differently, something that this book will seek to cover in depth. For starters, take the fact that for a woman, fasting is an easy way to throw your hormones into frenzy.

So how exactly does IF have to do with female hormones?

## The Intermittent Fasting-Hormone Connection in Women

By 'connection', we are simply alluding to hormonal imbalance.

Intermittent fasting can indeed cause hormonal imbalances in women. Unlike men, nature has conditioned women to be extremely sensitive to starvation signals. In a woman, if the body catches wind of starvation, it promptly kicks up the production of hunger hormones. This is why the moment many women break the fast, they face a seemingly insatiable hunger. This is your female body's way of shielding a potential fetus, and maximizing its chances of survival. This is the case even when you are not pregnant.

Before you assume ignoring these hunger cues will solve everything, consider this; the female body, when faced with multiple ignored hunger cues, may well respond by halting ovulation and leading to infertility. This is why women should ease their way into intermittent fasting. While there are no conclusive tests of this done on humans (and for obvious reasons), enough have been conducted on animals. In one study conducted on animals, after 2 weeks on an abrupt intermittent fasting program, menstrual cycles stopped in female rats. The ovaries shrunk and insomnia levels grew considerably high.

This is why the recommendation is, for one, to schedule your fasts so that you do it on non-consecutive days. By doing this, you get your body used to fasting so that over time, fasting becomes something your body is used to, and responds to positively.

I know you might be thinking, aren't you supposed to eat breakfast and 6 small meals that nutritionists recommend? Let's discuss that next.

# The Flawed Science Behind '6 Small Meals per Day

Why does every other book speak about '6 small meals a day'? In this chapter, we shall seek to understand the flaw in this thinking and then stack it against eating in specific windows.

Many diet books, manuals, and programs recommend 6 small meals a day. You are probably at odds with intermittent fasting given that it is impossible to work a 6-meal plan into the feasting window.

The 6-meal plan advice is one this chapter will examine. What arguments support the 6-meal plan? Are they viable? Is the science behind them scientific in itself? It is hard to make a case for it.

Here are several reasons why the 6-small meals a day plan thinking has flaws and why you should ditch it for intermittent fasting:

## Flawed Reason 1:

When you eat, your body has to burn extra amounts of calories just to complete processing this meal. The 6-meals a day reasoning comes from the theory that if you eat 6-meals spread across the day, your body will be constantly burning extra calories, keeping your metabolism firing at an optimal capacity.

This sounds quite practical, right? Well, this is far from the truth, and is mostly 'bro-science' that just does not hold up under real scrutiny. In truth, it does not matter if you spread 2,000 calories over your entire day or consume it in a small window: your body will burn the same number of calories when processing this food.

Thus, this argument of keeping your metabolism perpetually primed and working at optimal capacity only sounds good in principle. Reality tells a whole different story altogether.

## Flawed Reason 2:

When you eat smaller meals, you will be less likely to over-indulge.

This is partly true especially for those of us who struggle with portion control or have little idea of how much food we should be eating. Once you get used to intermittent fasting and the kind of responsible eating it inspires, you will properly understand just how much food you should be eating. You will also find out that the prospect of having 6 meals a day looks too prohibitive and exhausting. It is also not too far-fetched to think that with 6 small sized meals, you will probably never really feel full and will be very tempted to snack. In fact, given that 'small' is relative, every likelihood is that you are likely to eat a lot more calories only to end up gaining weight instead of losing it.

Although anchored in principles that appear quite logical, it is obvious that the 6-meal plan does not work for the reasons you would think it does. Also, as far as losing weight goes, it only really works for people with no portion control problems.

Think back to the caveman days. Our ancestors would have been in a lot of trouble if they had to eat every 3 hours. There is no way the human species would survive. Going further with this argument, it makes a lot of sense why the cave dwellers had very little trouble with stubborn body fat and obesity: they ate when they could, which was not too often, and their bodies adapted to this so that they used the food consumed in the most efficient way possible. This is the same logic intermittent fasting subscribes to.

With that understanding, let's now discuss the different ways in which you can follow intermittent fasting.

# Intermittent Fasting Protocols That You Can Follow As a Woman

## 1: The Lean-Gains Intermittent Fasting Method for Women

Started by Martain Berkhan, this type of intermittent fasting method is ideal for the woman who is open to exercising regularly in the gym and who is not only interested in losing weight, but also building some lean muscle.

### How the program works

You will fast for 14 hours a day. You can push this up to 16 hours, but the 16-hour fast is mainly for men.

You will then proceed to feed for the remaining 10 hours of your day. During the period of fasting, you are not to feed on any calories. There are exceptions to this, though. Black coffee is alright and may make the fasting period a bit more bearable. Calorie free sweeteners are also not a problem. If you can access sugar-free gum, it will also not mess up your program and will do good to keep you occupied. A bit of milk in your coffee will also do you no harm.

Your hours are your own and as such, this book can only recommend your fasting hours. It is however best to schedule your fasting period in a way that ensures the bulk of it falls in your sleeping hours. You will fast through the night and into your morning, terminating your fast about 6 hours after waking up.

This schedule should be easy to adapt to your schedule. However, understand that maintaining a consistent feeding window is important if this is going to work. Otherwise, especially as a woman, you risk throwing your hormones out of balance, and in the process, make it very difficult to adhere to the program.

What you eat and when you eat during your window of feeding should be reliant on when you exercise. On the days you exercise, carbohydrates should take precedence over fat. On the days you rest and do not hit the gym, fats should take precedence over carbohydrates. As for protein, your protein consumption should be quite high every day. However, this should vary according to your age, goals, levels of activity, and body fat. Regardless of all these things, you should make a point of avoiding processed foods. Your primary diet should consist of unprocessed foods.

There will be times when you do not have the time for a proper meal. At those times, rather than snack on unhealthy foods, keep a protein shake nearby. Keep it simple; powder and water protein shakes are often enough. If you cannot easily access this, which should be almost impossible if you live in the US, consider 'natural protein shakes' like eggs. A meal replacement bar is also acceptable. However, use the meal replacement bars in moderation.

## The Pros

The best thing about this program is that the meal frequency is irrelevant, which is good news if you are used to frequent snacking. If you want, you can break it up into 3 meals.

## The Cons

Even though the eating frequency is unchecked, there is close monitoring of what you eat. Processed foods are unacceptable. You will also have to eliminate conventional snacks and instead eat as much of veggies, fruit, and lean meat as you can since this sort of food works best with an exercise routine.

## 2: The Eat-Stop-Eat Fasting Protocol For Women

The brainchild of Brad Pilon, this intermittent fasting method suits women familiar with, and used to a healthy diet i.e. women who can adhere to a healthy eating diet.

### How the program works

You will have a 24 hour fast once or twice a week. During this aptly named '24 hour break from eating', you will consume no food. However, you can drink calorie free beverages. After completing the fast, you can then go back to your regular eating pattern. As Pilon says, "behave as though you did not fast at all."

It is also recommended that you arrange your fast so that immediately it is over, it is time for you to have a big meal, say, lunch or dinner. However, you can also schedule the fast to end in time for an afternoon snack. You should go with whatever works for you. As your schedule changes, you can adjust your timing.

What is the main rationale of this program?

Well, when you eat this way, you will able to reduce your calorie intake without having to put limits on what you eat. You simply target how often you eat as opposed to what you actually eat.

It is vital to note that when following this program, regular workouts, especially resistance training, will greatly help you realize your intended fat loss goals.

## The Pros of This Program

24 hours seems a long time to go without food. The good news is that this program offers you room for flexibility. On your first few weeks, you do not have to go all out and adhere to the 24 hour fast. In fact, on your first day, focus on going for as long as you can without food. You can then gradually build on this so that you steadily increase the number of hours you fast. Pilon recommends that you begin your fast on a day when you are particularly busy and are less compelled to break your fast.

The other benefit is that with this program, there are no forbidden foods. You will not count calories, weigh food, or place any restrictions on your diet. This makes the program a lot easier to follow than most. This said, it does not mean all kinds of food are allowed. As the founder says, "You still have to eat like a grown up." Moderation is important. A slice of cake is fine but going after the whole cake is not.

## The Cons

Going for 24 hours with no calories may be quite difficult for you. In fact, fasting for 24 hours straight can be brutal to sustain especially in the first few weeks, regardless of the flexibility the program offers you. It may not just be the battle of willpower giving you problems: your body could just as easily decide it does not like what you are putting it through and respond with symptoms such as fatigue, headaches, and high levels of anxiety.

# 3: The Crescendo Fasting Protocol for Women

This one is especially specific to women as it recognizes the very realistic danger of having unbalanced hormones courtesy of fasting. As such, it is not as intense or as demanding as the rest of the programs created to be viable for both men and women (typically, women fast for fewer hours in these programs.)

With crescendo fasting, you will fast on non-consecutive days. The name crescendo fasting comes from the fact that you will be gradually working your body until you can settle on a fasting approach that works for you.

## How Does Crescendo Fasting Work?

You will start with a 12 to 16 hour fast on 3 days a week. Just to make it clear, you will not do the 3 days of fasting in a row.

On these 3 days, you will focus on healthy eating during a restricted window. Your window could be, say, from 11 AM to 7 PM. You can easily achieve this by skipping breakfast altogether. If you are exercising as well as following the program, reduce your exercise intensity during the fasting days. Make the training sessions shorter by your standards depending on what your normal training routine looks.

One other thing that really helps, though not completely necessary, is BCAAs (branched chain amino acids). BCAAs will keep the protein building blocks in your system and prevent muscle breakdown. However, the biggest benefit, as far as BCAAs go, is that when you supplement with them, they greatly mitigate the insatiable hunger many women experience especially in the first several weeks of adopting this fasting protocol.

*Briefly: Fast on 2 to 3 non-consecutive days*

On your fasting days, do yoga, light cardio, or strength training. The objective is to keep the training routine mild. Ideally, you should fast for 12 to 16 hours.

On the days you perform hard exercises like high cardio, eat normally. High cardio exercises are activities such as hours-long running, metabolic conditioning, biking for long hours, and the likes.

During your fast, you should strongly consider taking about 8 grams of BCAAs

Take plenty of water during your fasting period. Coffee and tea with a little milk in them are not bad as well

After 2 weeks, feel free to add 1 more day of fasting

**Tip**: If you are still tentative about intermittent fasting, start out with this program as it is somewhat less demanding than the rest.

# 4: The Warrior Diet Intermittent Fasting Protocol for Women

Started by Ori Hofmekler this dies is ideal for women who have an ironclad discipline and do well with following the rules. This fasting protocol is intense, perhaps more than the other programs. It is suitable for you if you are looking to drop weight as quickly as possible. It is also ideal for women under 35.

## How the Program Works

You can expect to fast for 18 hours every day and only eat one large sized meal at night. What you eat as well as when you eat your large meal is vital in allowing this program to work for you.

The philosophy adopted by this program is to have you feed your body the nutrients it needs in synchronization with the 'circadian rhythms'. It also builds on the theory that dating far back to the caveman years, humans were primarily nocturnal and as such, inherently programmed for nighttime feeding.

You may have guessed, and rightly so, that a 20 hour fast every single day without eating anything is too brutal and unrealistic. The fasting phase here is not about shutting yourself from food entirely: it is really more about under-eating.

During your 20 hour fast, you can eat veggies, several servings of fruits and protein, and even fresh juice. This is supposed to optimize the SNS's (Sympathetic Nervous System) 'fight or flight' response. This response promotes body alertness, stimulates fat burning, and boosts your energy.

Ori Hofmekler calls the 4-hour window the 'overeating phase.' It falls at night to optimize the Parasympathetic Nervous System's capacity to aid your body recuperate and in so doing, promote calmness, relaxation, and digestion. At the same time, it allows the body to use up the nutrients consumed for its growth and repair. According to the founder, eating at night may also stimulate your body to produce hormones that help it burn body fat in the daytime.

During the 4-hour eating window, the order in which you eat food groups matters a lot as well. You should start with veggies, fat, and then protein. After you eating these groups of food, you can eat some carbohydrates. However, you should only eat the carbohydrates if you still feel hungry.

## The Pros

Many people have chosen this program because the fasting period allows you to snack. This makes it easier to get through.

## The Cons

While it is certainly nice to snack during the fasting hours, it is quite rigid especially in relation to what you can eat as well as the order in which you can eat it. The schedule is strict and the meal plan is, as you can see from the 'how the program works' paragraph, tightly controlled.

You can adopt a wide variety of intermittent fasting protocols. However, the question remains, which is the most suitable fasting window. Let us find

# Which Fasting Window Is Beneficial To You?

Having learned the different intermittent fasting methods, it is also critical to know the best fasting window so that you can gain the most from intermittent fasting since after all, you are adopting intermittent fasting to lose weight.

Ideally, you should be able to fast for 12-16 hours without any issues. This means that you can do the Lean-Gains and crescendo fasts. Simple, right?

Not so fast! There is the controversial issue of your body going into survival mode. Your body does this for self preservation. Thus, if you spend more than 14 hours without food, your body starts storing up any food it gets instead of burning fat. This is definitely not good for weight loss.

So, what should you do?

You need to reprogram your body as it were. Start training it to understand that it is not in danger of starvation. This means fasting for 12 hours 3 times a week to begin with. This is why the crescendo method is quite popular. It allows you to build up to your fasting hours. If you fast for 12 hours, you can fast from 8pm-8am. This means that you will be able to eat 3 meals or more during the feeding window.

However, you must not forget your goal.

Your goal is weight loss. If you fast for only 12 hours, you are just giving your body enough time to enter into the fasted state where fat burning occurs. This means that if you eat after just 12 hours, your body will only be able to burn a bit of fat. That's not very practical, is it? You want to burn as much fat as you safely can. This means increasing the number of hours you will be in the fasted state.

Since your body is just getting used to fasting, you should increase your fasting window to 14 hours. This is just enough time to allow your body to burn fat without triggering the starvation mode. Start by fasting for only 3 days in a week. If you have your last meal at 8pm, you can have your first meal at 10am. It is not that hard.

Gauge your body to see how you feel. As you get more comfortable, you can increase your fasting days. You can move from the crescendo fasting method to the Lean-Gains one with little difficulty. However, remember to keep your fasting hours to 14 hours only. Try as much as possible to keep regular fasting hours.

As the weeks go by, you will lose weight even if you rarely exercise. But once you reach closer to your ideal weight, you'll find yourself 'stagnating' at the same weight measurement. This is normal. This is the time to think seriously about exercising and keeping fit. This is the time to watch what you eat.

## So, what should you eat?

Basically, when you adopt intermittent fasting, you should be able to eat whatever you want. But as we know, not all foods are equal. Some are better for you than others are. Thus, your fast should resemble something like:

Saturday night at 8pm: Eat your last meal of the day.

Saturday at 10pm: Go to bed as usual. This means you would have already fasted for 3 hours.

Sunday morning at 7am: Wake up and start your day. By this time, you've fasted for 11 hours.

Sunday 7am-10am: You only spend 3 hours fasting while you're awake.

Sunday 10am: Eat your first meal of the day.

You will have a 10-hour feeding window. Your meal plan can be:

Breakfast: cottage cheese, Greek yogurt, almonds and berries

Lunch: salad greens, chicken and avocado

Dinner: sweet potato, steak and veggies

The idea is to eat more vegetables, fruits and protein and less carbohydrates. Don't worry so much about counting calories. You just need to be conscious about reducing the amount of carbs, you eat and the rest will take care of itself.

Once you lose weight, you can then employ other fasting methods such as the warrior diet or the eat-stop-eat methods. This will just be to help you maintain the weight loss. You can also decide to just stick to the 14-hour fast if you wish as it works very well and it has very few rules.

I believe you now have a clear understanding of how to follow intermittent fasting as a woman. Next, we will discuss strategies that will increase your odds of success.

I believe you now have a clear understanding of how to follow intermittent fasting as a woman. Next, we will discuss strategies that will increase your odds of success.

# How To Adopt Intermittent Fasting And Maximize Effectiveness Of The Fast

This chapter has tips to help, especially if you are relatively new to fasting. If you follow them, you will have a much easier time fasting and will be able to incorporate it into your social life as well.

## Do Not Freak Out

Too many newbies freak out over all sorts of details. Stop obsessing over things such as "whether it is ok that you only fasted 15 hours instead of the recommended 16 hours." Also, eating an apple during your fasted period will not ruin everything. You need to relax!

Your body is not some tool that is powerless unless you carry out everything to perfection. If there was a fine piece of machinery, your body is it. Your body can adapt to just about anything.

If you feel like eating breakfast today and do not feel like it tomorrow, this is just fine.

## It Is Okay If People Give You Funny Looks From Time To Time

You will likely have a few people who will look at you funny when you tell them you fast, or you no longer eat breakfast. How can you be normal if you do not have 3 meals a day? Explaining things to them will not help much; it is easier to just smile and let it go. Embrace it and keep going.

## 'Commit Excessively'

This may seem a bit counterintuitive, but your best intermittent fasting plan should see you start on a day when you are incredibly busy. Do you have a day scheduled when you will be working multiple hours on a major project? Schedule your fasting period to start on this day. It will be much easier to get through it compared to starting on a day when you are lazy and more likely to want to snack.

## Zero Calorie Beverages Are Fine

Really, they are. Just because your program wipes breakfast off your plate does not mean you cannot have a kettle of green tea to help with your morning duties. If you want to drink water, tea, or black coffee during your fasted periods, it is okay. The key thing is to keep things simple and not overthink if you want to be in fasting for the long haul.

## Ensure you stay hydrated

This is common sense: staying properly hydrated will make your fasting periods a lot easier to live through. When you drink a lot of water, you will feel satisfied since your belly will have something in it. This will pare the edges of your hunger pangs. In addition, many people confuse thirst for hunger; therefore, when you feel hungry, just take a glass of water and you will feel much better.

The amazing thing about water is that it not only manage hunger but also helps flush out toxins.

Water is especially important because it not only reduces hunger but it also helps flush out the toxins in your body. If you're hungry, drink a glass of water. More often than not, people confuse thirst with hunger. Once they drink a glass of water, they find that they were not as hungry as they thought. Drinking water will keep your body rejuvenated throughout the day.

## Fast Overnight

You do not have to follow this one. It helps though, if you choose to. Make an effort to fast through the night. You will likely not be done with the fasting period by the time you wake up, but you will have at least slept through 8 or so hours of your fasting period.

Another thing you can do is eat your dinner earlier than you are used to. This will lengthen your 'night hours' such that you won't have to wait for long before eating breakfast. For example, if you eat your dinner at six and you need to fast for fourteen hours, you can have your breakfast at eight. This makes intermittent fasting achievable for more people as it is within their reach. The more you normalize intermittent fasting, the easier it becomes for you to achieve it.

## Lock down your kitchen

As you start intermittent fasting, it would be good to remember that hunger can be deceptive. Here is the thing. You eat because your body needs fuel in order to carry out various functions. This fuel can be sourced from three places. These are carbohydrates, fats and proteins. When you are fasting, your body still has all the fuel it needs for you to engage in various activities, as it burns fat. This means that there is no need for you to keep eating when you already have the fuel you need.

This may be easier said than done.

If you're used to eating 3-6 meals per day, you may find it a bit difficult to adjust to the diet. One thing you can do is make it a bit harder to get to the food. You can have lockdown periods whereby you lock down your kitchen during your fasting window. Place some post-it notes on the door to remind you why you are doing the fast. Also, remind yourself that food will still be waiting for you at the end of your fasting window. This will help you stick to your fasting pattern as your body adjusts to the new pattern of eating.

## Eat well but don't overindulge

It would be good to remember that intermittent fasting is a deliberate action. Yes, your body goes into fasting mode. However, it is also assured of getting nourishment after a certain period. This means that you should not eat food as if it is going out of stock. Of course, you may find yourself eating a little bit more. However, there is a difference between eating until you're full and eating for the sake of eating. If you are feeling full, stop eating and wait for the next feeding window.

Once your fasting period is over, prepare the food, set the table and sit down to eat. You should eat slowly and deliberately. This means putting down your fork between bites, chewing your food properly and interacting with your companions during the meal. The idea is to fully enjoy the meal and avoid gulping it down simply because you are fasting. If you take your time to eat your meal, your meal, your brain will know that everything is okay and there's no need to panic as the food is available when you need it.

## Revise Your Thought Process

This means you must stop viewing fasting as some sort of less-than-desirable process you have to get through. Simply think of fasting as taking a break from eating. Think of it as an opportunity to take away the constant worry of what you are going to eat next or what will be in the different meals in your day.

This kind of mindset is uniquely powerful. Suddenly, the fasting period will not be something you are dying to get through so you can hit the fridge. Your fasting period will be somewhat like a period of meditation: a period of calm and purity that allows your mind to be free of worry. Think of the fasting period as an unperturbed stretch of time where you can work in peace. When you do not have to get up constantly to fix up some meal, you can do more and focus better.

## Go To The Gym

When you fast intermittently and combine it with gym work, you will experience better results and will shed body fat faster. You do not have to be obsessive with your gym work: a few minutes on the treadmill, or a few body weight exercises will be enough.

When you follow all the above guidelines, you should definitely expect a number of benefits.

# The Benefits: What To Expect

In this chapter, we shall seek to understand the potential health benefits of intermittent fasting.

Let us start with the potential benefits you stand to enjoy when you fast intermittently:

## 1: Intermittent Fasting Changes Cellular, Genetic, and Hormonal Function

When you do not eat for a while, a few things usually happen in your body. For instance, your body will initiate important cell repair processes and changes in the hormonal levels all shifts, which serve to make stored body fat a lot more accessible to the body to convert into energy.

When you fast, here are a few changes that will occur in your body:

1. Insulin levels in the blood drop considerably thus facilitating the fat burning process

2. The levels of growth hormone in the blood may increase up to 5 times. High levels of growth hormone usually facilitate fat burning, and offer a host of other benefits

3. The body often induces vital cellular repair processes, which include the removal of waste products in the cells

## 2: It Will Help You Lose Weight and Stubborn Belly Fat

The truth is that most people who try intermittent fasting do it in a bid to lose weight. Toward this end, intermittent fasting anchors on a very simple, straightforward principle: you eat less frequently, which leads to fewer meals and fewer calories. Unless you compensate by eating an unusual amount of calories during your eating window, or focusing on foods rich in simple carbs, the guarantee is that you will end up eating fewer calories.

In addition, as you may have picked up from the first point, intermittent fasting will enhance hormonal function in a way that facilitates weight loss. Lower levels of insulin, higher levels of growth hormone and higher levels of noradrenaline will all facilitate the process of breaking body fat for energy production.

## 3: Slows Down Aging and Helps Fight Various Diseases

They say age is just but a number. But when signs of aging set in, especially for women, this brings with it lots of stress, fears, and lots of other negative feelings. The immediate response is to apply lots of makeup and use various procedures to hide the signs of aging but as you well know, this is only temporary and outward; if you are aging, you will feel it on the inside. That's why you need a solution that actually works on your body to help it fight/reverse aging.

Intermittent fasting is a great solution for slowing aging, as it inhibits the cellular pathway known as the mTOR, which is responsible for aging from performing its functions.

More conclusions have also been drawn around the connection between toxins/dead cells accumulation and diseases. It has been seen that IF helps clear toxins in the body; the toxins that are at the core in promoting illnesses. This in turn minimizes the positive impact that toxins have on your overall health. Essentially, this 'clean up' of toxins aids the body to resist illness and promotes physical agility. You feel refreshed and energized after toxins cleanup.

This also promotes mental clarity, heart health, reduced cancer risk and outwardly, a beautiful beaming skin.

When talking of increasing lifespan and IF, simple conclusion applies. If your chances of suffering heart problems and getting cancer are reduced by whatever percentage, that is a likelihood of compressed morbidity, a less likely chance of dying from those diseases and thus a plus to the age limit.

## Caveat – Not All Should Really Fast

Expectant, lactating, diabetic and hypoglycemic individuals should not fast. If you are pregnant, please do not fast at all, at least for now. This is because of the energy requirements you currently have to sustain your gestation period. The same applies to breastfeeding mothers.

Diabetes (high blood sugar) and hypoglycemic (low blood sugar) diseases are also prohibitive to any form of fasting. This is because of the insulin and glucagon control issue that is mainly anchored in glucose control and you do not want to alter it further by fasting.

# How To Avoid Muscle Buildup

Unlike men, most women striving to lose weight are never keen on any muscle toning. Instead, a beaming skin in a slender agile body flaunting long hair is the ideal setup. Nonetheless, it is important to keep in mind that during fasting, that is the period of lowest insulin production. In that case, chances of muscle build up and general body mass increment are high. The reason boils down to how hormones ability to impact on energy conversion is normally at peak during periods of starvation.

*In order to comprehend this muscle build up during fasting consider this:*

Naturally, when there is less food intake and thus less energy supply, the body must utilize the stored energy. Glucagon in effect helps to convert stored glucose (glycogen and fats) to energy. The first energy requirement in the body is to the muscles, where physical energy source is. Therefore, the first set of glycogen to be converted to energy is that stored in the muscles. That explains why physical ability is the first to deplete during starvation and the first energy supply soon after food intake is to the muscles also. At the same time, the first and the most vital energy storage need is still to the muscles. This makes it easy for muscles to bulge very easily soon after fasting ends especially if feasting is accompanied with heavy work outs.

Therefore, a secret to avoiding muscle buildup for women during IF is to keep vigorous physical activity to the lowest during the whole period of fasting and feasting.

## The HGH effect

Yet another hormone contradicting the preferred state of affairs in women is the growth hormone, the HGH. What the hormone does essentially is to encourage cells and tissues growth. This can easily result in muscle growth.

However, if you do not want too much muscle, first, understand that you cannot control or suppress the secretion of this hormone; you can only work around it wisely by minimizing its effects. See tips below:

- Remember that light duties are physically less demanding. Stick to them and avoid extensive workout that might stimulate muscle buildup.

- Abstain from attempts of eating during the fasting window. This starves the HGH of any glucose and its effects on growth are therefore negligible. Without any glucose coming, the growth hormone will have to compete for the glucose converted from stored glycogen and other energy sources e.g. any proteins converted to glucose, as well as fats, a factor that also accelerates fats breakdown.

- Approach the intermittent fasting formula subtly. Start with shorter fasting regimes as you progress to a full one like a 24 hours window to allow your body to gradually adjust to energy production and conversion rates.

# I Need Your Help...

We have come to the end of the book. Thank you for reading and congratulations for reading until the end.

As you have found out, intermittent fasting is truly a smart way to lose weight and attain many other benefits. Moving away from the 6-meals a day dogma and being able to replace it with something less demanding is so relieving. Additionally, with intermittent fasting, you do not have to count calories. You can choose to, if you want, but you do not have to.

Ladies, if you are sick and tired of all the quick fixes supposed to transform your life and yet, only make you progressively weaker, if you want to gain the multiple benefits of intermittent fasting, feel good, and like what you see in the mirror, you need to start fasting intermittently.

Now that you have read this book, you can go about fasting in a smart way.

Finally, if you enjoyed this book, then I'd like to ask you for a favor, would you be kind enough to leave a review for this book on Amazon? It'd be greatly appreciated!

I want to reach as many people as I can with this book, and more reviews will help me accomplish that!

Thank you and good luck!

# Preview of 'Anti-Inflammatory Diet Guide'

## Effects Of Inflammation

Inflammation is the biological response your body goes into when dealing with harmful stimuli such as irritants, pathogens or even damaged cells. It is a self-protection mechanism that allows your body to begin the healing process. The 'hotness' or 'inflammation' you feel after you cut yourself or injure yourself is the result of your body working hard to heal itself. But what happens when your body experiences 'too much' inflammation?

A little inflammation is not a bad thing. In fact, when it happens, you should rejoice in knowing that your body is working tirelessly to correct the situation. However, like most good things, inflammation can get out of hand. When this happens, you may experience various health complications such as:

## Weight Gain

Every day, thousands of people try to lose weight to no avail. They complain that they've tried out various diets but somehow none seem to be working. If they do find something that works, sooner than later, they are back to gaining the weight they thought they'd lost. This is because they neglect to look into inflammation as the cause for their weight gain. Inflammation contributes to weight gain in various ways. These include:

- If inflammation happens in the brain, it interferes with the functioning of the hypothalamus and this in turn increases your appetite and slows down your metabolism. When this happens, you will be eating a lot but burning up less energy, which leads to weight gain.

- Gut inflammation leads to leptin and insulin resistance. Leptin is the satiety hormone that tells your brain when you have had enough. When suffering from leptin resistance, you just eat and eat some more before leptin can communicate that you have had enough, which leads to weight gain. Another thing that gut inflammation does is to increase intestinal permeability. When this happens, more toxins will be able to permeate your bloodstream. Usually toxins are stored in fat cells to remove them from circulation. The more toxins you have, the more the fat cells expand to accommodate the more toxins leading to weight gain.

- Inflammation in the endocrine system suppresses adrenal and thyroid function. One of the main functions of the adrenal gland is to burn fat. Therefore, when you suppress the functioning of the adrenal gland, you are unable to burn fat, as you should leading to weight gain.

As you have read, inflammation is bad for you if you want to maintain the ideal weight.

## Metabolic Syndrome

Metabolic syndrome refers to a group/cluster of lifestyle-related diseases including cardiovascular disease and obesity. They are clustered together because all of these diseases are linked to metabolic dysfunction. Markers of metabolic dysfunction include:

- Central obesity – this is excessive tummy fat

- Hyperinsulinaemia – this refers to ongoing high levels of insulin

- Insulin resistance –your body loses sensitivity to insulin (you need more insulin to manage your blood sugar levels)

But the question is how these three factors are connected. Well, when on a diet high in carbohydrates, your blood sugar levels increase leading to high insulin levels to help blood cells absorb the glucose and thus manage your blood sugar levels. When you have high insulin levels, the production of cytokines (which are pro-inflammatory) increases and in turn this causes inflammation especially in predisposed persons. Once inflammation increases, it brings with it an increase in the production of free radicals. Free radicals affect cellular functions and one of those functions just happens to be insulin sensitivity. This is why chroni low-grade inflammation is linked to all three markers; that is, raised insulin levels, obesity and decreased insulin sensitivity.

## Chronic Fatigue

Many people suffering from chronic fatigue have been told that the disease 'is all in their minds'. Fortunately, in recent years more researchers have began looking into the association of chronic fatigue and inflammation. This is mainly because the two possess many similar symptoms including muscular pain and tenderness, sore throat, joint pain, swollen lymph nodes and sore throat.

As you know, inflammation is the way your body reacts to foreign particles. When you have symptoms of inflammation, it is safe to say that your body is fighting something even if that something is not yet known. This is why researchers link an overactive immune system to chronic fatigue.

Another thing that associates chronic fatigue with inflammation is the lack of cortisol in patients suffering from chronic fatigue. Cortisol is known to suppress inflammation. Thus, if your body has a cortisol deficiency, it will not be able to suppress inflammation and this will worsen symptoms of chronic fatigue. A dietary change often helps people suffering from chronic fatigue.

## Some types of arthritis

When you hear the name arthritis, you automatically associate it with pain. Well, it is no coincidence since arthritis refers to inflammation in joints. When your joints experience inflammation, you will feel pain. The types of arthritis that have been linked to inflammation include:

- Gouty arthritis

- Rheumatoid arthritis

- Psoriatic arthritis

- Systematic lupus erythematosus

When you suffer from these types of arthritis, you may experience inflammation symptoms such as redness, joint stiffness, swelling of the joints, pain in the joints and loss of joint function.

It is important to note that inflammation does not have to be painful for it to be present. This is because many organs in your body just don't have enough pain-sensitive areas for you to feel that inflammatory sensation. This means that you can suffer from chronic inflammation over time without knowing, only for you to experience the effects of inflammation.

It is also important to note that various things can cause inflammation including:

- Processed foods high in sugar and unhealthy fats

- Omega-6 fats (and not enough Omega-3 fatty acids)

- Sleep deprivation

- Chronic stress

- Smoking

- Pollution

- Environmental chemicals

- Lack of exercise

Thus, chances are, if you experience any of the above things, you may be suffering from inflammation whether or not you experience pain.

The first thing you should do once you notice that you suffer from inflammation is not to reach for drugs because drugs just address the symptoms and not the root cause but rather to make some lifestyle changes. This is because most of the causes of inflammation can be addressed by making lifestyle changes like exercising more, reducing exposure to pollutants, not smoking and dietary changes.

In this book, we will focus on addressing inflammation by adopting an anti-inflammatory diet. Let us learn more about anti-inflammatory diet in the next chapter.

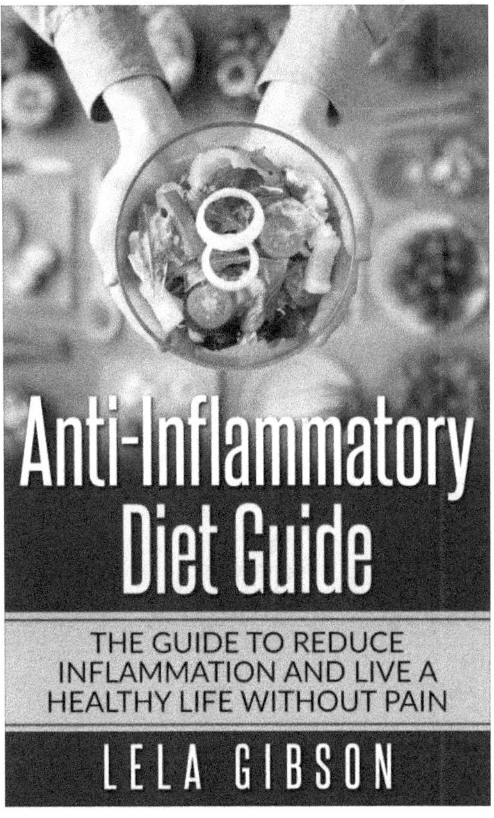


**Check out the rest of Anti-Inflammatory Diet Guide on Amazon, go to: http://amzn.to/2qKTSPa**

# Check Out My Other Books

Below you'll find some of my other popular books that are popular on Amazon and Kindle as well.

Alternatively, you can visit my author page on Amazon to see other work done by me.

**Ketogenic Cookbook: Quick Low Calorie Ketogenic Crockpot Recipes with 7 Days Meal Plan**

**Freedom: How to Make Money Online and Become Financially Free by Creating Passive Income**

**Mediterranean Diet: Instant Pot Cookbook with Delicious Recipes**

**Alice the Superbug**

**Madison and Astrid's first magical journey**

**Intermittent Fasting: The Essential Beginners Guide for Women for Weight Loss**

**Chakra Healing: Chakra Healing and Karmic Awareness for Beginners**


**SEO 2017 for Growth: The Ultimate Guide to Learn Search Engine Optimization with Internet Marketing Tips**

**Psychology: How to Analyze People Using Human Psychological Techniques, Body Language Signals, Social Skills and Personality Types**


**Paleo Smoothies: Recipes to Energize and for Ultimate Health and Weight Loss**


**Belly Diet Smoothies: Delicious Smoothie Recipes to Flatten Your Belly, Improve Your Gut & Burn Fat**

**Keto Diet: Keto Diet Guide Cookbook for Beginners with Meal Plan and Simple, Delicious Recipes to Lose Weight and Look Good**


**Online Business from Scratch: The 9 Step Guide to Building a Profitable and Sustainable Online Business**

**Weight Loss: 20 Easy And Fast Diet Tips For Losing Weight - An Easy-To-Follow Weight Loss Guide**

**Ketogenic Cookbook: Ketogenic Cookbook for Beginners with 7 Days Meal Plan**

**Negative Calorie Diet: Cookbook & Guide Which Will Help You To Burn Body Fat, Lose Weight And Live Healthy**

**Negative Calorie Diet with Anti-Inflammatory Diet Guide**

**Make Money Online To Achieve Freedom**

**Negative Calorie Diet with Smart Fat Guide**

**Negative Calorie Diet & Clean Eating: Cookbook & Guide Which Will Help You To Burn Body Fat, Lose Weight And Live Healthy**

**Smart Fat: Cookbook with Fat Meals Which Help You to Lose Weight, Get Healthy and Improve Brain Function**

**Anti-Inflammatory Diet Guide: The Guide to Reduce Inflammation and Live a Healthy Life Without Pain**

**Essential Oils: The Young Living Book Guide of Natural Remedies for Beginners for Pets, For Dogs**

**Clean Eating: Cookbook and Guide to Restore Your Body's Natural Balance and Eat Healthy**

**Anti-Inflammatory Diet Guide: The Guide to Reduce Inflammation and Live a Healthy Life Without Pain**

**Dash Diet: Cookbook for Weight Loss with Action Plan and Easy Recipes**

**Air Fryer Cookbook: Quick, Healthy and Easy Low Carb Air Fryer Recipes**

**Psychology & Habits Of Highly Effective People Box Set**

**Leptin Resistance: Leptin Diet to Control Your Hormones, Get Permanent Weight Loss, Cure Obesity and Live Healthy**

**Negative Calorie Diet & Dash Diet Box Set**

**Negative Calorie Diet & Weight Loss Box Set**

**Habits of Highly Effective People: What Are the Habits of Successful People?**

**Slow Cooker: Cookbook with Slow Cooker Recipes**

**Weight Loss Cookbook: Meal Prep Cookbook for Weight Loss and Clean Eating**

**Weight Loss Cookbook: Mediterranean Diet for Lasting Weight Loss**

**Negative Calorie Diet & Dash Diet Box Set**

**Slow Cooker & Instant Pot Box Set**


**Children Books: Madison and Astrid's first magical journey & Alice the Superbug Box Set**


**Belly Diet: The Zero Belly Diet Step-By-Step Guide Which Helps You to Lose Your Belly and Enjoy Your Flat Belly**


**Weight Loss: 20 Easy and Fast Diet Tips for Losing Weight - An Easy-To-Follow Weight Loss Guide**


**Instant Pot: Instant Pot Pressure Cooker Cookbook with Easy and Healthy Recipes**


**Vegan Cookbook: Vegan Cookbook For Beginners, For Kids And For Teens For Diabetics With Pictures**


**Low Carb: Low Carb Diet Cookbook with Low Carb Keto Recipes for Batch Cooking**


**Ketogenic Cooking: Ketogenic Cooking With Your Instant Pot**

**Passive Income: Passive Income Tutorial with 7 Online Ideas to Generate Passive Income Streams for Beginners**

**Low Carb Diet: Low Carb Diet Recipes Cookbook for Beginners for Batch Cooking**

**Make Money from Home: How to Make Money Online and Escape the 9-5 Rat Race**

# Bonus: Subscribe To The Free Weight Loss Report

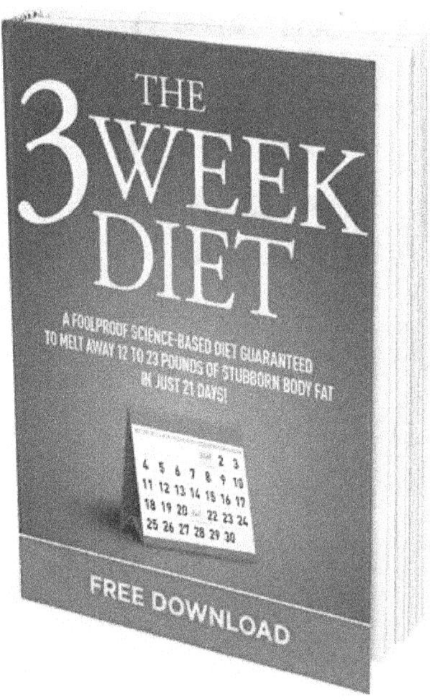


The Introduction Manual is more than just an introduction to the diet. Instead, it discusses the science behind how we gain and lose weight as well as what absolutely needs to be done to attack that stubborn body fat that, until now, has been so challenging to get rid of.

Here are the preview of what you'll get:

- Rapid Weight Loss

- How This System Works

- Why This Diet

- Why 3 Weeks?

- 21 Days To Make A Habit

- Fat Loss VS. Weight Loss

- Nutrients

- Protein, Fat, Carbohydrates

- The Food Pyramid And Obesity

- Fiber

- Metabolism

- How We Get Fat

- Triglycerides

- How To Get Thin

- Diet Overview

- Meal Frequency

- Water

- Diet Essentials

- Let's Get Started

To get instant access to these incredible ebook, go to:
http://bit.ly/2tUb9cp

www.ingramcontent.com/pod-product-compliance
Lightning Source LLC
Chambersburg PA
CBHW070044260726
48658CB00002B/721